DIY: HOMEMADE MEDICAL FACE MASKS

A STEP BY STEP GUIDE WITH ILLUSTRATIONS TO PROTECT YOU AND YOUR FAMILY WITH CUSTOM FIT FACE MASKS

MAGDA HEWITT

Copyright © 2020 by Magda Hewitt

All rights reserved.

No part of this book may be reproduced in any form or by any electronic or mechanical means, including information storage and retrieval systems, without written permission from the author, except for the use of brief quotations in a book review.

CONTENTS

1. Introduction	1
2. Medical Masks and Why we Need Them	5
3. Important Factors to Consider When Making The Masks	11
4. Tools Required	17
5. Taking Custom Measurements	19
6. Drafting Your Pattern	27
7. Preparing your Fabric	39
8. Assembling your DIY Medical Face Mask	45
9. Additional Safety Precautions to Observe	59
10. Cleaning your Face Mask	63
Afterword	65

1
INTRODUCTION

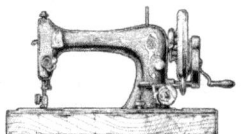

The current crisis that the world is experiencing has led to a massive shortage of medical masks. Never in the history of the world has this been experienced, we are literally all in this together.

In an ideal world, it would have been great to get access to respirators or even commercial medical masks, but we are living in unusual times.

This book aims to teach you how to make your own, custom-made mask, for yourselves and your family, thus helping to solve the problem of the mask shortages, currently being experienced worldwide.

You could also make masks and help others by donating

them to people in need of masks, and those who do not have access or the means to get one.

I am currently making masks and donating them to the nursing homes in my area, as a way of giving back.

I am a full-time fashion designer, specializing in wedding and evening wear. I made my first face mask when a client of mine approached me, freaked out over the fact that masks have been sold out in local stores.

That is when I realized there is a huge need for people to learn how to make their own masks. Since then, I have been doing a lot of research as to what kind of fabrics would be suitable to use, as well as how to make a mask that will keep me and my family safe and protected.

I will not bore you with the various kind of fabrics and their efficacy, but for this book, I'm working with 100% cotton, tightly woven,) as it seems to be one of the safest options, fabric wise.

Various patterns can be used, but I've found the pattern I'm going to teach you to be the best. It fits properly, as it's custom made, and it severely limits any bacteria or viruses from entering through the filters.

This book guides you and teaches you how to make a mask from home that fits you properly, protecting yourself and your family.

This DIY tutorial guides you, helping you make a four-layered medical mask, with one layer being a pocket to hold a removable filter, should you be able to get a hold of one.

Here is what you can expect to learn from this book:

- The importance of a face mask.
- Understand which fabrics are best to use for face masks, and why.
- Learn how to take custom measurements to ensure a snug fit that molds perfectly around the chin, nose, and jawline.
- Design your custom face mask pattern.
- You will learn how to assemble your face mask with a sewing machine. All sewing can also be done by hand. It takes a bit longer, but that how our ancestors learned to sew, and they did just fine.
- The importance of additional safety protocols when wearing your face mask.
- Maintenance and cleaning your mask.

The following two chapters briefly explain the importance of a face mask and show you the tested effectiveness of various fabrics. This will help you make an informed decision when designing and creating your mask. We then look at all the requirements you'd need in order to make your mask. I include professional materials and provide you with everyday alternatives as well. (We don't all have access to a French curve ruler or an over-locker.)

Finally, I will teach you how to make your own custom-fit medical face mask.

I'm going to try to make the tutorial as simple as possible. Literally, anyone can learn to do this. While most of the fabric mentioned can be bought from your local fabric store, the idea is that you can still use everyday household fabrics. Within the suggested guideline, I will teach you which standard household fabrics are the most effective and can be used, even if you cannot get to a local fabric or a haberdashery store.

2
MEDICAL MASKS AND WHY WE NEED THEM

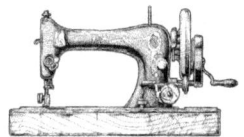

Would the usage of masks help curb the spread of the current pandemic?

That is the golden question, and perhaps the biggest reason why people have been buying medical masks in bulk. This surge of medical mask purchases has resulted in numerous governments pleading with the public to stop buying masks. With ordinary citizens buying out all available masks, there is a shortage of them. First responders and the sick people who need them the most are suffering because there is simply not enough. Suppliers also seem to be struggling to keep up with the demand.

I don't want to bore you with the history of pandemics or

masks, as most of us are feeling a bit overwhelmed with the news coverage every day.

This book is to help you learn how to make an easy yet effective mask that can offer some protection. You'd get to spend some time with the family and kids, teaching them a skill while bonding. Learning this essential skill might help in restoring some sense of control in our lives.

Before starting, there are a few basic things you need to understand.

To understand the importance, or rather, the value of a medical mask, it's essential for me to mention the two main types of medical masks briefly.

1. Surgical Masks

These masks, also commonly known as medical masks, can generally be bought from your local pharmacy or ordered online. They are loose-fitting and disposable after a single-use.

It is not advisable to wash and reuse store-bought surgical masks, as the effectiveness of these masks is then drastically reduced.

While there are several surgical mask options, including homemade options, a good surgical mask should have a minimum of three filter layers to ensure effectiveness.

While these masks offer a certain level of protection, they

are not safe for medical staff to use around infected patients. The reason for this is because these masks are designed to hold out larger airborne droplets, but tiny particles can still filter through them.

2. Respirators

Currently, the respirator is the preferred mask used by healthcare professionals when dealing with infected patients, because of the mask's ability to capture even the tiniest of particles.

This is the more effective solution as these masks help protect against airborne viruses, smoke, dust, air pollution, and, depending on the mask, help block out vapors and gasses.

The most popular of these masks used in the medical field are respirators.

Respirators holds out up to 95% of virus, dust, and pollution particles. This refers to the tiniest of particles, and should, in theory, even offer you protection from larger particles like life-sized bananas.

> *PRO TIP: If you find yourself in a situation where life-sized bananas are flying around in the air, ducking is probably your best bet.*

The above information is just for some general basic knowledge, regarding the most-used mask today. Now, when you hear these terms mentioned on the news, you can have a basic understanding.

Our focus is on creating a mask that can provide you with some form of protection against infections and you spreading the infection to someone else.

Why do we need medical masks?

There is a common misperception that masks are intended for the safety of the person wearing the medical mask.

While medical masks do offer a certain level of protection, the real protection is for those around you. The medical mask is mostly intended to protect people around the mask-wearer from his or her respiratory emissions.

When we wear a mask in public, we are not only protecting ourselves but those around us. Likewise, when the people next to us wear a mask, they are protecting us.

When you look at it that way, you realize that wearing a mask is an act of kindness. When people around you wear masks, they protect you, and you, in turn, reciprocate that kindness by doing likewise.

It's pretty uplifting when you look at it that way.

Benefits of making your own mask

1. You can ensure that the mask fits you properly, as the pattern is custom made to your facial measurements. Most store-bought masks are made to standard face sizes, hence the reason some don't fit properly. The correct fit is essential, as it should fit as snugly around the face as possible, to prevent any germs and viruses from passing through.

2. It's something that can be done with the kids. During this stressful time, kids can be taught a skill, and it allows for some bonding time away from the daily stresses we're currently experiencing.

3. By creating your masks, you won't need to resort to hoarding medical supplies, relieving pressure on the medical health professionals that need these supplies the most.

Many factors need to be taken into consideration before making a mask. There is a lot of information out there on making quick, five-minute masks. However, the reality is that merely layering paper towels and tissue paper is not sufficient enough to ensure your safety and the safety of those around you.

In the following chapter, we will look at crucial factors you need to consider when making a mask.

3
IMPORTANT FACTORS TO CONSIDER WHEN MAKING THE MASKS

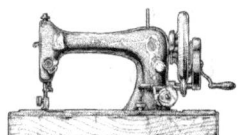

There's a lot of conflicting information available on the web. Some of that information even claims the effectiveness of ordinary rolled up toilet paper, held onto the face with an elastic. While a lot of these measures do offer some protection, the key question remains:

What can I use to make an effective homemade face mask?

To answer this question, we need to look at two critical aspects of the mask.

Effectiveness of a mask

There are two important factors to consider when determining what fabric to use when creating your mask. Knowing the research behind the different types of fabric is important when deciding what fabric to use.

1. Breathability

It's simply not practical creating a mask that can capture a high number of particles if you cannot breathe through it. You would have to continually lift your mask to take in a gulp of air, which defeats the purpose of the medical mask.

2. Particle capture

The most effective mask can filter out a very high percentage of particles.

So, What fabric is the best to use when creating a mask? We don't want to suffocate while wearing it, but we also need it to be as effective as possible.

To answer this question, Cambridge University[1] completed a study in 2013, where they tested how effective different types of materials were at capturing tiny particles.

The tests included a range of household fabrics that could be used as an effective mask filter. They tested a variety of products ranging from a vacuum cleaner bag, dish towels, cotton shirts, and even woolen scarfs.

The scientists tested the efficiency of each fabric against 0.02-micron bacteriophage particles. (For us non-scientific folk, basically these particles are five times smaller than the Coronavirus.)

A single-layered store-bought surgical mask performed the best, being able to filter out up to 89% of these particles. Coming in a close second was the vacuum bag at 87%. Although, I'm not all that keen on sticking a used vacuum bag around my nose.

The single-layered dish towel managed to filter out an impressive 73%. The cotton-blend pillowcase at 61% and the cotton shirt at 51%.

These results are great, but since most decent masks have at least two layers of filters, the researchers decided to double each of these items and test for effectiveness.

A double-layered medical face mask was able to filter out 97% of the particles. Perhaps even more impressive is that a standard household, double-layered dishcloth could also filter out up to 97% of the tested particles.

The effectiveness of a double-layered cotton shirt increased to 71% and a double-layered cotton-blend pillowcase increased to 62%

. . .

Based on the above results, the solution is simple, right? Make a double-layered dish cloth mask, or perhaps even the vacuum bag, since both offer a whole lot of protection.

Except, the researchers have selected 100% cotton and cotton-blend pillowcases as the preferred choice for a homemade mask.

Why on earth would they do that? Surely, the cotton options are not as effective, and so it doesn't make sense using these options?

The answer to that question lies in the breathability of the fabric. While the double-layered dishcloths are effective filters, the fabric itself has very little breathability.

This is the reason why I would suggest you use layered cotton fabric when making your masks. The cotton should preferably be 100% cotton. Ideally, the higher the thread count of the cotton, the better. With an increased thread count, your fabric would be able to filter out more, while ensuring you can still breathe.

In this book, we use three layers of cotton fabric to help keep you protected and ensure you can breathe in the process.

Now that we have discussed the best fabric to use when making homemade medical face masks, and more importantly, *why* they are the best, the next chapter quickly goes over the tools required to make your face mask.

---

1. https://smartairfilters.com/en/blog/best-materials-make-diy-face-mask-virus/

4

TOOLS REQUIRED

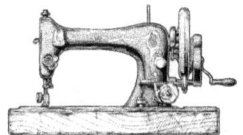

I'm a full time designer, but I understand that not every one has access to interfacing, a French curve ruler, or even a sewing machine. The good news is that you don't need all the fancy equipment to make your mask.

I will provide you with a list of requirements you'd need in order to get started. I will also provide you with a list of common household items you can use as alternatives.

Requirements to make your own mask

1. Sewing Machine. Your mask can also be sewn by hand if you do not have a sewing machine, although it will take a little longer.
2. A pair of scissors. If possible, use one scissor to

cut out the paper pattern and another to cut out the fabric.
3. A tape measure.
4. Three A4-sized pieces of paper. We will be drafting our patterns on paper.
5. Fabric. I will be using 100% tightly woven cotton, washed. You can also use good quality bed sheets, or pillow cases if you can't get to a fabric shop.
6. Thin elastic string for the ear-loops. I'd suggest a 1/4 inch width if possible.
7. Pins. If you do not have pins, you can use a small weight to hold down the fabric.
8. Pencil.
9. Straight ruler, or anything to draw a straight line with. You could even use your measuring tape if you do not have a ruler.
10. A French curve ruler. If you do not have access to this, don't stress. You can manually draw the curve when we design our pattern.

5

TAKING CUSTOM MEASUREMENTS

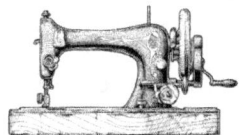

*S*tore bought surgical masks are made in standard, one-size-fits-all. This results in a loose fit, particularly around the edges.

A key component to a good, quality mask is that it filters out as much as possible. With that reasoning, having open edges does not help with keeping you protected.

An efficient mask should fit securely around your face. It doesn't help having a material that is able to filter out a high number of particles, but still has openings for viruses and bacteria to enter.

I will be teaching you how to make a custom-made face mask

that fits snugly on your face. The most important step in any custom measurement is learning how to take accurate measurements.

To make the face mask, five measurements are required.

We will be doing a sew-along with this tutorial. The measurements I will be using for the purpose of demonstration in this book is my son's exact measurements.

You will need to use your own measurements.

You will be given a guide on how to take your measurements.

Before we begin drafting our pattern, you need to have the measurements at hand.

Use the below format when jotting down your measurements:

Measurement 1 – Mid-nose tip to side face, stopping an inch away from the ear.
(Insert your measurement)
Measurement 2 – Upper bridge of nose to the tip of the nose.
(Insert your measurement)
Measurement 3 – Tip of the nose to below the chin.
(Insert your measurement)
Measurement 4 – Upper bridge of nose to the chin.
(Insert your measurement)

Measurement 5 – **Length of ear measurement.**
(Insert your measurement)

Details for each measurement can be found below, with illustrations to show you how to take each measurement.

For the sake of this tutorial, I will be making a face mask for my son and so all the measurements will be his. These measurements simply serve as a guide, and your measurements will differ depending on who you're making the mask for.

Measurements required

Measurement 1

Mid-nose tip to side face, stopping an inch away from the ear.

My measurement is 4.5 Inches/11.40 cm

Write down your measurement. You will use this when drafting your pattern.

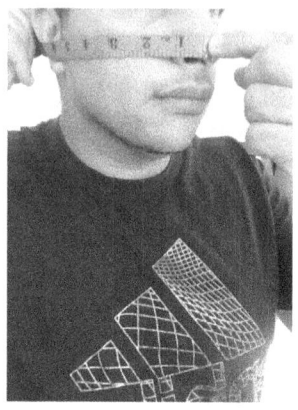

Measurement 1

Measurement 2

Upper bridge of nose to the tip of the nose.

My measurement is 1.5 Inches/3.80 cm

Write down your measurement. You will use this when drafting your pattern.

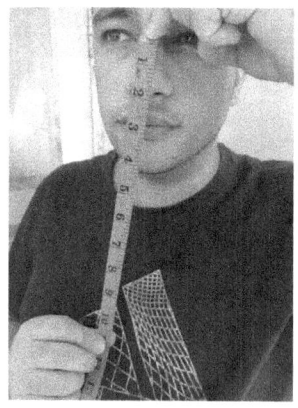

Measurement 2

Measurement 3

Tip of the nose to below the chin. (Where the mask should end)

My measurement is 4.5 Inches/11.40 cm

Write down your measurement. You will use this when drafting your pattern.

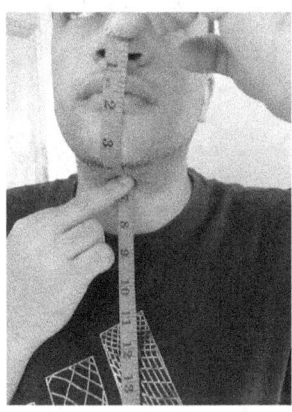

Measurement 3

Measurement 4

Upper bridge of nose to the chin. (Where the mask should end)

My measurement is 6.5 Inches/16.5 cm

Write down your measurement. You will use this when drafting your pattern.

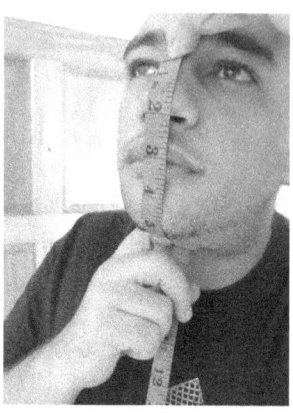

Measurement 4

Measurement 5

Length of ear measurement. (This will be used for the side of face measurement.)

Note: This measurement is taken to give you a rough guide on how wide the sides of your mask should be. Thumb-sucking the width of the mask might cause gaping — this measurement is to help prevent that.

My measurement is 2.25 Inches/5.6cm

Write down your measurement. You will use this when drafting your pattern.

Taking Custom Measurements | 25

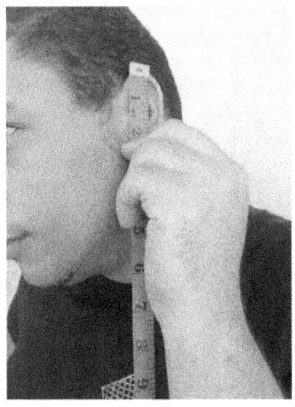

Measurement 5

DRAFTING YOUR PATTERN

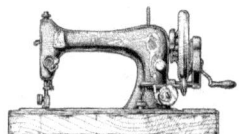

The mask I'm going to design is based on my son's measurements from the previous chapter. The idea is to give you a draft along experience to help you make it yourself, with your own measurements.

The drafting of the pattern will be divided into three separate parts to help you follow along easily. To draft your pattern, you will need the measurements taken in Chapter five.

We will also be labelling each Point in the pattern so that you can easily follow the instructions.

PART 1

Step 1.

Draw a square on a piece of paper equalling 8 by 8 inches.

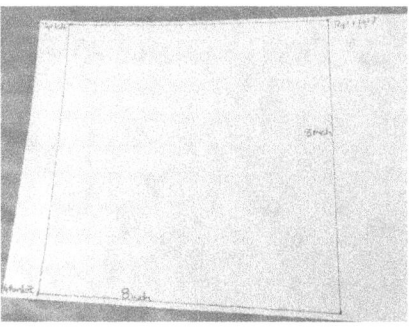

Step 1

Step 2.

Locate the top left corner of your square and mark it 'A.'

Step 3.

From Point A measure **down** 1.5 inches
 Note: This will be measurement no. 2.
 You will use your own measurements for this step.
 Pencil a mark and label that 'B.'

Step 4.

From Point B, go down by another 0.5 inches and make a mark. Label that 'C."

Note: The 0.5 inch allowance is so that the mask will not fit too tightly around the nose.

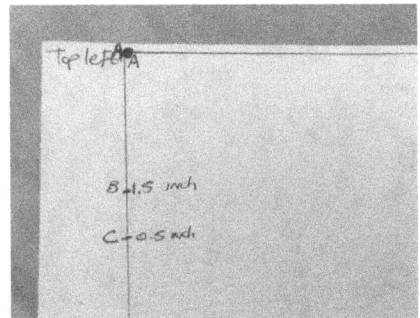

Step 2, 3, and 4

Step 5.

Find the mid-point between B and C. Label that D

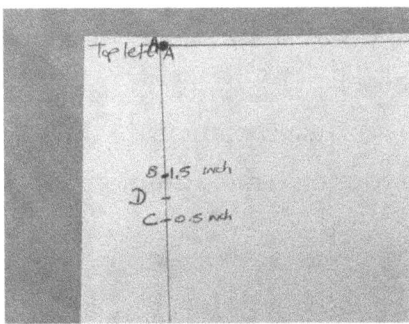

Step 5

Step 6.

Ensuring that the ruler is straight, draw a straight line from Point D across to the right side of the square.

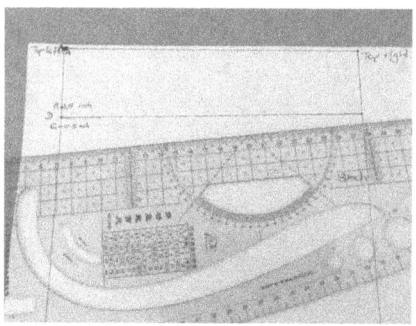

Step 6

Step 7.

From Point A, go down by 6.5 inches and make a mark, labelling that Point E.
   NOTE: This is measurement no. 4
   You will use your own measurement for this step.

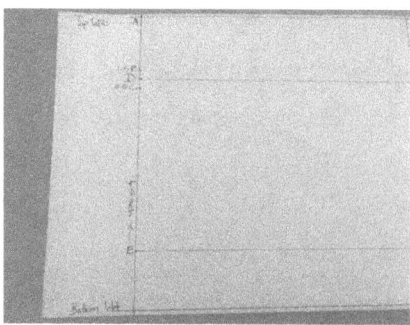

Step 7

Step 8.

Ensuring that the ruler is straight, draw a straight line from Point E across to the right side of the square.

Step 9.

From Point E move across to the right by 1.5 inches and make a mark. Label this Point F.

Note: The 1.5 inches is a standard allowance for adults, done to give shaping to the lower face area. Adjustments can be made later.

If you are making the mask for a child, the allowance should be 0.75 inches instead of 1.5 inches.

The 1.5 inches as shown below is for an adult.

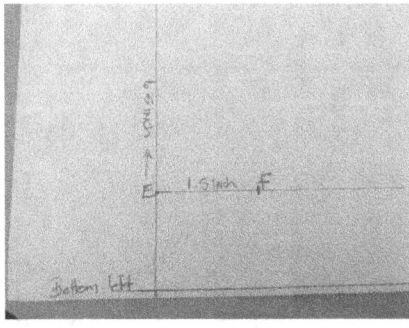

Step 9

Step 10.

From Point A move across 1.25 inches and make a mark. Label this Point G.

Note: The 1.25 inches is a standard allowance for adults, done to give shaping to the bridge of the nose area. Adjustments can be made later.

If you are making the mask for a child, the allowance should be 0.5 inches instead of 1.25 inches.

The 1.25 inch allowance as shown below is for an adult.

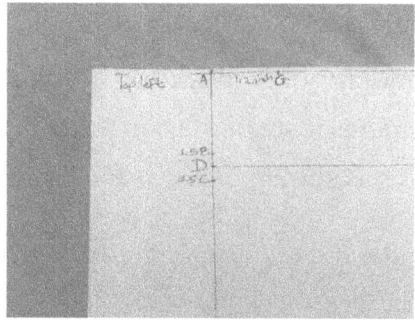

Step 10

Step 11.

From Point D move across by 4.5 Inches and make a mark. Label that Point H.

NOTE: This is measurement no. 1.

You will use your own measurement for this step.

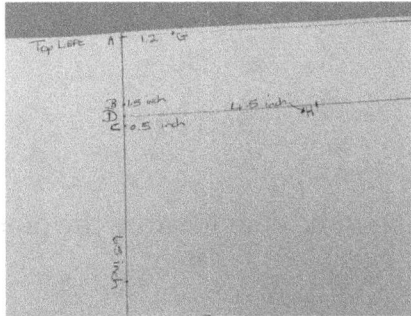

Step 11

Step 12.

Take measurement no. 5 (Length of ear measurement.) and draw a vertical line on Point H as shown in the below illustration.

Your measurement's midPoint will rest on Point H.

In my case, the ear measurement is 2.25 inches.

Label the one end of the ear measurement Point I and label the other end Point J.

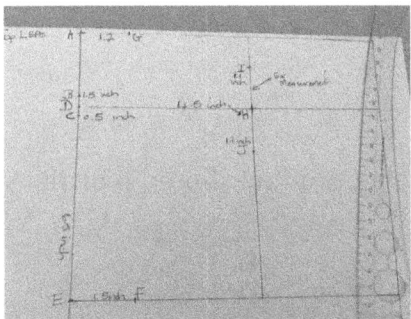

Step 12

PART 2

Now we are going to start connecting the points made in the steps above.

Connect all the marks as per the below instructions.

Step 1.

Draw a straight line from Point I to Point G.

Step 2.

Draw a straight line from Point G to Point B.

Step 3.

Draw a straight line from Point C to Point F.

Step 4.

Draw a straight line from Point F to Point J.

Your completed product should look like this:

Drafting Your Pattern | 35

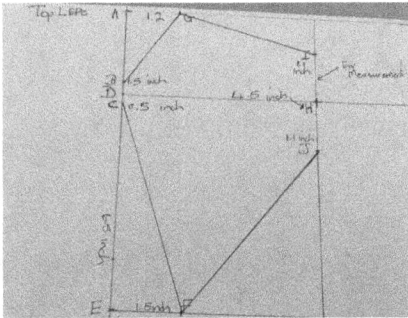

Step 1, 2, 3 and 4

Part 3

Now that we have drawn our lines, we can begin shaping our mask.

Step 1.

Find the midPoint between F and J. Mark a Point and label it Point K.

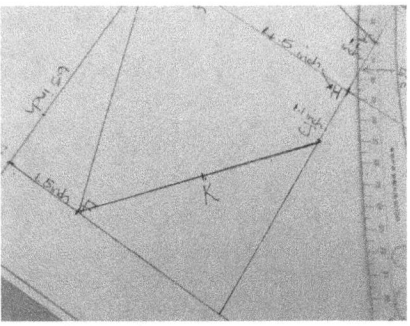

Step 1

Step 2.

Go in by a quarter inch from Point K. Make a mark on your pattern.

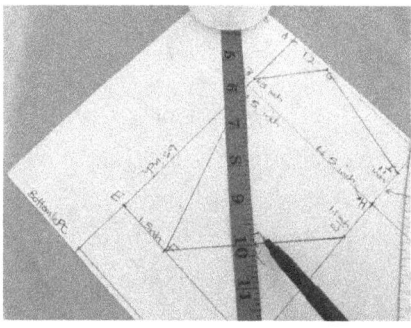

Step 2

Step 3.

Use the mark made in step 2 as a midPoint and draw a curve from Point F to Point J. This is to assist with the fit around the cheeks.

You can use a French Curve ruler for this step, but you can also draw the curve manually by hand.

Drafting Your Pattern | 37

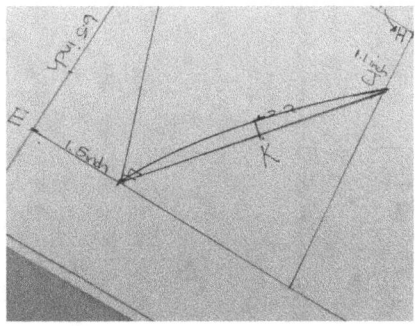

Step 3

Step 4.

Repeat the above steps for Points I to Points G.

Find the mid-point between I and G. Make a Point. Mark that Point L

Step 5.

Go in by a quarter inch from Point L. Make a mark.

Step 6.

Use the mark made in step as a midpoint and draw a curve from Point I to Point G. This is also to reduce excess fabric under the eyes.

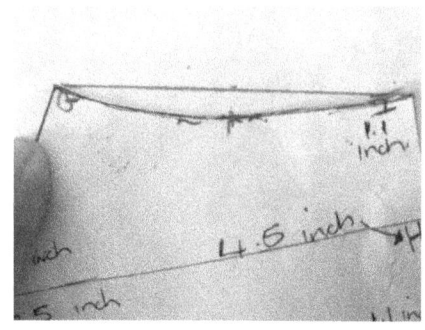

Step 6 - Your curve can also be drawn by hand

Step 7.

Shape the curve between Point B and C. This step will help prevent Pointed edges around the nose.

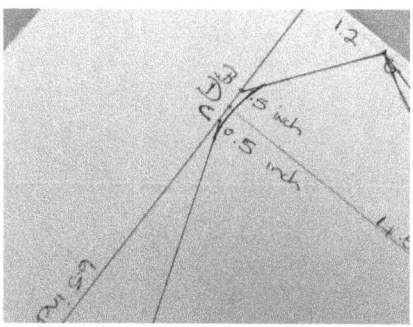

Step 7

PREPARING YOUR FABRIC

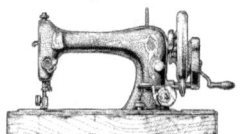

We will now use our pattern to cut out our fabric.

NB: If this it brand new material, it is important to wash your fabric for the first time before making your mask. If you make the mask and wash it afterwards, you will not have a perfect fit because the fabric will shrink.

PART 1

Step 1

You will need eight layers of fabric, roughly 2 inches larger than your actual pattern.

40 | DIY: HOMEMADE MEDICAL FACE MASKS

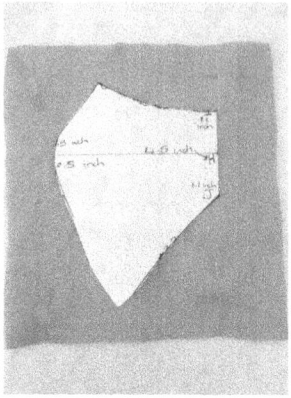

Step 1

Step 2

Take four layers of fabric and pin the pattern down onto the fabric, allowing a bit of fabric for a small seam allowance. The seam allowance will be 0.5 inches.

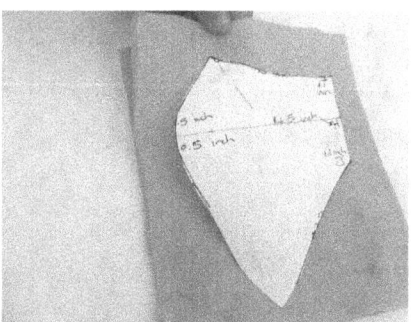

Step 2

Step 3

Trace around the pattern piece, allowing a 1 inch allowance on the side as per below illustration:

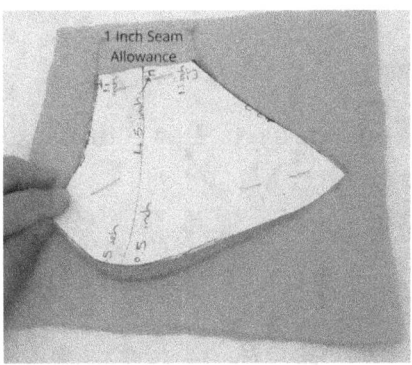

Step 3

Step 4

Cut out the pattern piece, allowing a 0.5 inch allowance

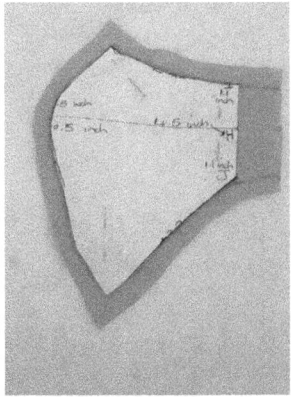

Step 4

Step 5

Take the cut out pattern and pin it onto the remaining four fabric pieces.

Step 6

Cut out to the same size as the first four pieces.

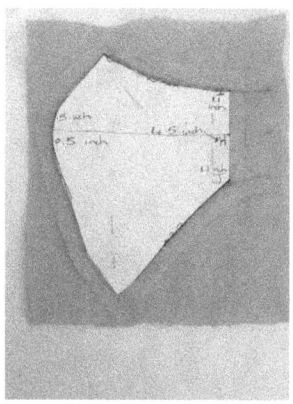

Step 6

Part 2

We will now set aside fabric to create our filter pocket.

Step 1

Remove two layers of the cutout fabric.

Step 2

Adjust the sides by 1.5 inches going inwards and draw a straight line as per below illustration:

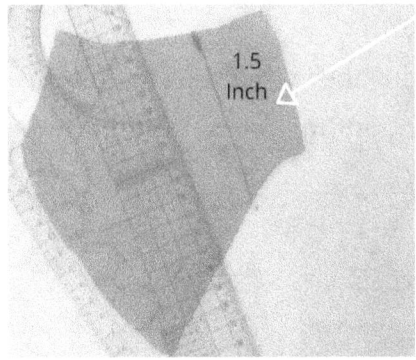

Step 2

Step 3

Cut off the excess fabric at the straight line.

By the time your fabric is cut out, your fabric pieces should match the below image:

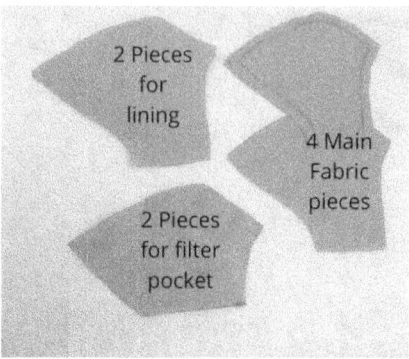

Step 3

Please use the above image as a reference point for when we start stitching our masks in the next chapter.

ASSEMBLING YOUR DIY MEDICAL FACE MASK

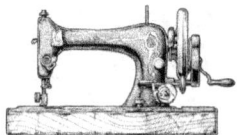

For the purpose of this tutorial, I will be using a dark sewing thread, so that you can clearly see the stitching lines.

Ideally, you would need a sewing machine to sew the mask, but it can also be sewn by hand, using a needle and thread.

We will begin by assembling the four main pieces of fabric.

PART 1

Step 1.

Taking the four pieces of fabric for the outer layer of the mask, pin them together as shown below:

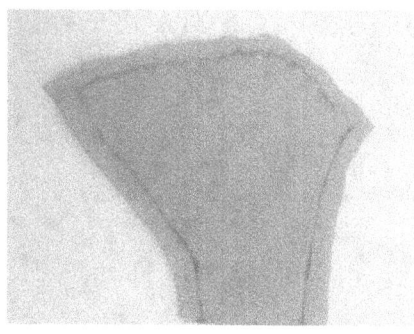

Step 1

Step 1

Step 2.

Stitch along the pins, following the 0.5 inch seam allowance.

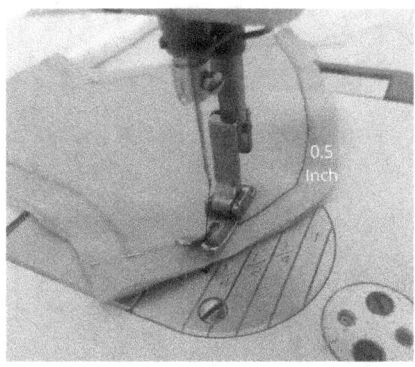

Step 2

Step 3.

Take the two pieces labelled lining, pin them together, following the 0.5 inch seam allowance.

Step 4.

Stitch along the pins

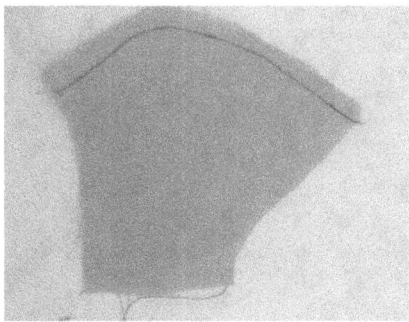

Step 4

Step 5.

Pin pocket filter pieces together at 0.5 inch seam allowance

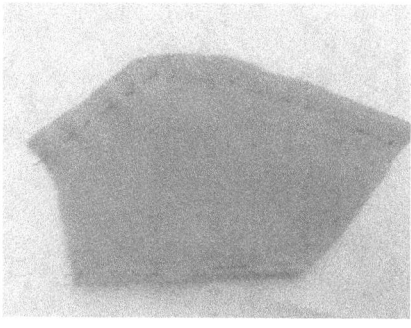

Step 5

Step 6.

Pin down the sides with a 0.25 inch allowance

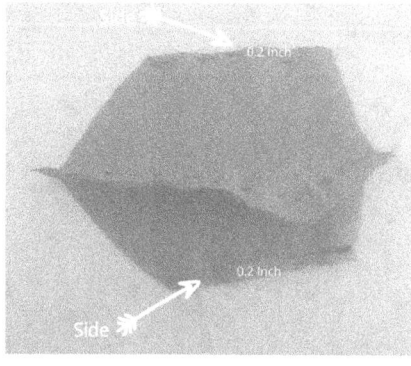

Step 6

Step 7.

Stitch the pins along the middle, joining both pieces.

Step 8.

Stitch along each of the sides, following the pins

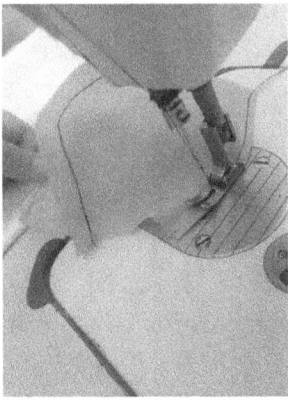

Step 7 and Step 8

PART 2

Now we will join all the stitched fabric pieces together.

Step 1.

Starting with the four main fabric pieces, make at least six small cuts along the edges as per below illustration.

Note: The nipped edges helps to shape the fabric

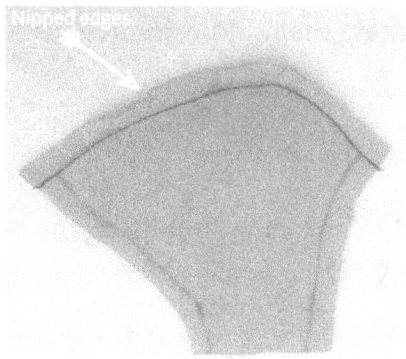

Step 1

Step 2.

Do the same for the remaining two pieces.

Step 3.

Open the seams on the main fabric and top stitch as per the three images below:

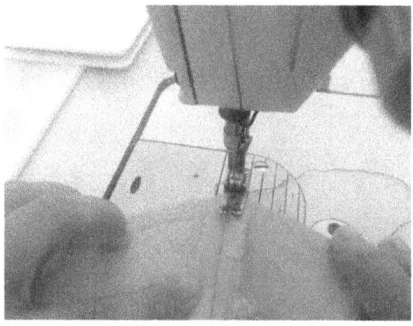

Step 3

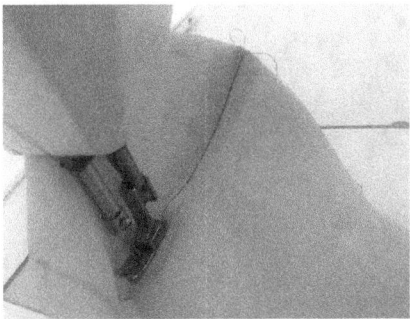

Step 3

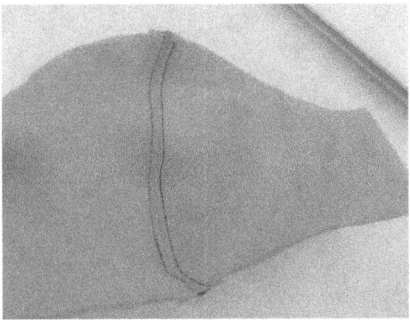

Step 3

Step 4.

Repeat step 3 for the lining and the pocket filter. (Open seams and top stitch)

Note: Top stitching is not necessary, but it does give the seams a neater finish.

Step 5.

Iron all the top stitched seams

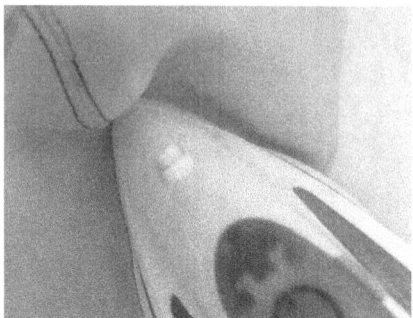

Step 5

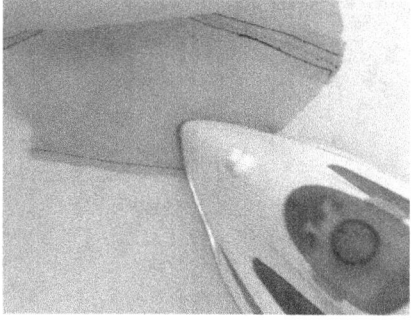

Step 5

Step 6.

Place the pocket filter onto the lining as per the two images below :

Assembling your DIY Medical Face Mask | 53

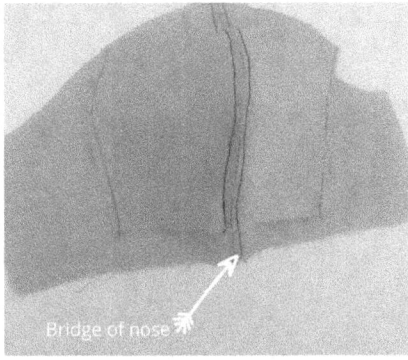

Step 6

At this point, fit the mask to face and see if any adjustments need to be made; meaning whether you need to loosen or tighten the mask either at the bridge of the nose or the chin.

Step 7.

Take the main fabric and pin it to the lining and filter pocket as per below:

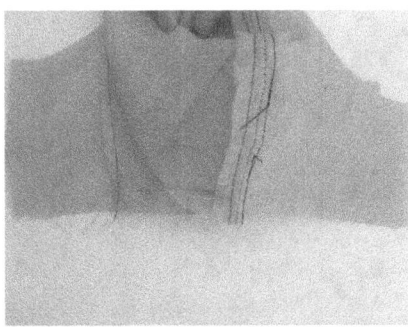

Step 7

Step 8.

Pin fabric pieces right around the edges at 0.5 inch allowance, leaving the sides open.

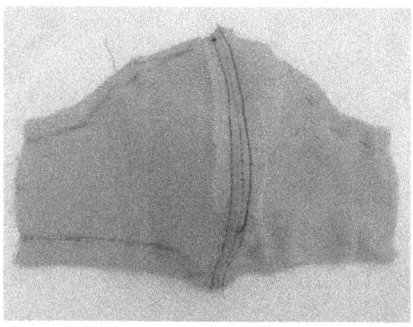

Step 8

Step 9.

Stitch along the pins

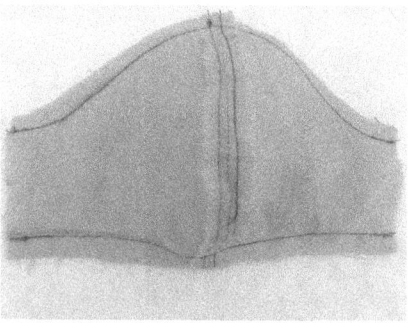

Step 9

Step 10.

Turn fabric inside out

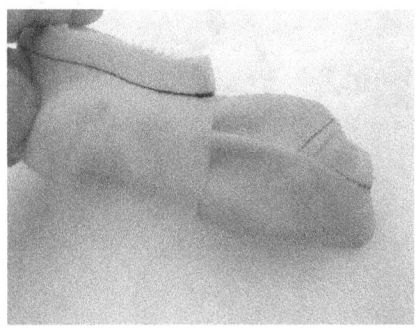

Step 10

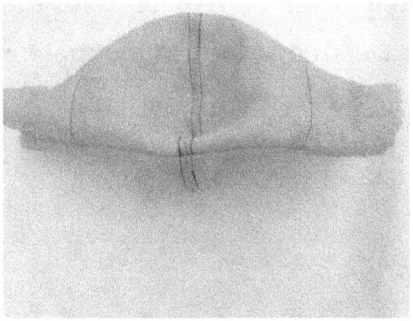

Step 10

Step 11.

Iron edges flat

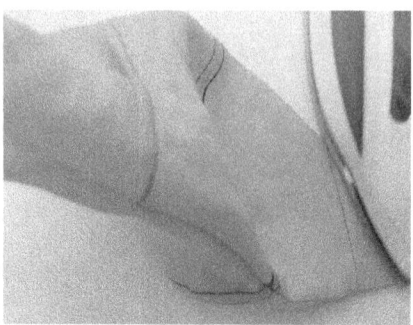

Step 11

Step 12.

Turn in the side edges by 0.5 inches, pin them up and top stitch. Be sure to leave enough of a gap for the elastic.

NB: If you have an overlocker or a machine that can do a zig-zag stitch, use those stitches to neaten the edges. For the purpose of this tutorial, I am simply going to fold and top stitch.

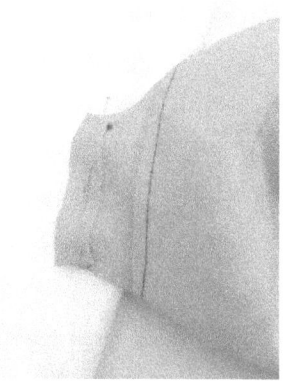

Step 12

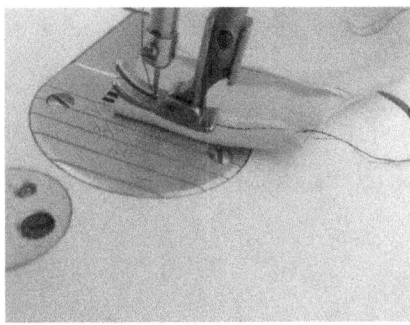

Step 12

Step 13.

Insert elastic string through both side openings, as shown in the picture below. I've used a safety pin, but you can also use a piece of wire to pull it through:

The length of the string for children is roughly 4 inches, and 8.5 inches for adults. Adjust elastic length accordingly as needed.

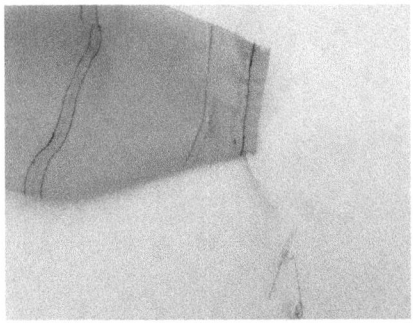

Step 13

Step 14.

Tie elastic strings, making a tight double knot.
Pull the knot to the insides so that the knot is hidden.

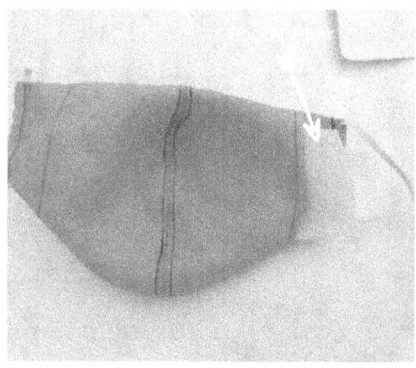

Step 14

And now you have your very own mask :)

9
ADDITIONAL SAFETY PRECAUTIONS TO OBSERVE

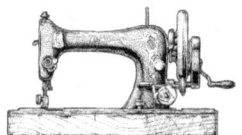

While your homemade mask certainly helps to protect you and those around you, it's important to remember that these masks can only do so much. Using the masks will help, in conjunction with these extra precautions to be taken.

Social Distancing

These words have become the new normal for humanity. Keep a safe distance from people around you.c The majority of infections happen when people are within six feet of each other. That is why we are all advised to stand a few feet apart from each other in public places. Too close contact with people can lead to contracting airborne illnesses.

Drink water regularly

If you are like me, then drinking water can be a major hassle. But health experts have advised that we should aim to take a sip of water every fifteen minutes. Even if the virus enters your mouth, the water washes it down to your stomach, and the acids inside your stomach can help kill the virus. If the virus enters your mouth and you do not drink enough water, it can quickly enter your windpipes and into your lungs. That is when it becomes dangerous.

Drinking warm water is useful for all viruses. Make it a habit to start drinking at least three glasses of hot water every day to help flush out any toxins in your body. Now is the best time for us to all aim to drink those eight glasses of water.

Keep warm

Keeping warm is especially essential when going outdoors. The Coronavirus is NOT heat resistant. A temperature of only 27°C/81°F would kill it. This also means that the virus hates the sun. This also explains why healthcare professionals suggest you drink warm water.

Personal Hygiene

The virus can only live on your hands for a maximum of ten minutes. But a lot can happen in those ten minutes. You could touch your eyes, nose, or mouth. Be sure to wash your hands with an alcohol-based sanitizer or soap as frequently as you can.

Gargling with a simple salt and water solution is useful as well. Mix a teaspoon with half a glass of warm water and incorporate gargling into your morning routine.

Avoid Metal surfaces

If the virus drops onto a metal surface, it lives for a minimum of twelve hours. Therefore, when you come into contact with any metal surface, be sure to avoid any contact with your face and wash your hands straight away.

Keep your clothes clean

The virus can last for roughly 6-12 hours on fabrics. Thankfully, your ordinary laundry detergent can kill it. After leaving the house, be sure to change into a fresh change of clothes and wash the clothes that could potentially have been exposed to the virus.

What to look out for to ensure you do not have the Coronavirus?

Many people start worrying about having been possibly infected once certain symptoms appear. What are the signs to look out for? when should you seek medical attention?

While I'm not a medical health expert, I can still share some of the research I've done with you.

If you have a runny nose and sputum, you most likely have a common cold. Coronavirus infected patients generally have a dry, painful cough with no runny nose.

If you start experiencing difficulty in breathing, it is imperative that you see a healthcare professional right away.

Majority of Coronavirus patients do not display any symptoms for up to fourteen days. This makes it difficult to determine whether you're infected or not, and by the time we land up in the hospital, it could be too late.

For this reason, experts have suggested a simple test that can easily be incorporated into your routine.

Take in a deep breath of air each morning and hold your breath for ten seconds. After ten seconds, slowly exhale.

If you can hold your breath successfully for ten seconds, this proves that there is no fibrosis on the lungs. In laymen's terms, there is no infection on the lungs.

If you are unable to hold your breath without coughing or major discomfort, seek medical attention immediately.

10

CLEANING YOUR FACE MASK

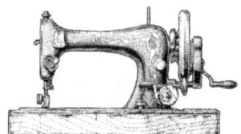

The face mask that we've just designed and sewn is a re-useable/re-washable medical face mask. It can only be used for between two–five hours at a time.

I would strongly suggest not using it for a period longer than that.

The effectiveness in the protection the mask will offer decreases due to the moisture from coughing, sneezing, and breathing into the mask. When fabric becomes wet, it loses its ability to filter.

For this reason, I recommend you make more than one mask per family member if possible, so that you can always have a backup mask should the other mask need to be cleaned.

Two to three masks per family member would be ideal. Carry a spare mask with you, storing it in a clean safe storage container, for when you plan on being outdoors for more than two hours at a time.

Your homemade DIY face mask can be reused many times, provided that you look after it.

The mask should be hand washed separately, with warm water. Normal detergent or even soap will do. Do not wash you mask with your other clothing. Ensure you wash it gently so as not to damage the fabric.

Once the mask is washed, hang it outside to dry.